INCREDIBLY DISGUSTING DRUGS

STEROIDS AND YOUR MUSCLES
The Incredibly Disgusting Story

Albert Spring

the rosen publishing group's
rosen central
new york

Published in 2001 by The Rosen Publishing Group, Inc.
29 East 21st Street, New York, NY 10010

First Edition

Library of Congress Cataloging-in-Publication Data

Spring, Albert.
Steroids and your muscles: the incredibly disgusting story / by Albert Spring. — 1st ed.
p. ; cm. — (Incredibly disgusting drugs)
Includes bibliographical references and index.
ISBN 0-8239-3393-8 (library binding)
1. Anabolic steroids—Health aspects—Juvenile literature. 2. Doping in sports—Juvenile literature. [1. Steroids. 2. Drug abuse. 3. Athletes—Drug use.] [DNLM: 1. Anabolic Steroids—adverse effects—Popular Works. 2. Substance-Related Disorders—Adolescence—Popular Works. 3. Muscles—drug effects—Adolescence—Popular Works. WM 270 S769s 2001] I. Title. II. Series.
RC1230 .S67 2001
615'.773—dc21
00-011987

Manufactured in the United States of America

CONTENTS

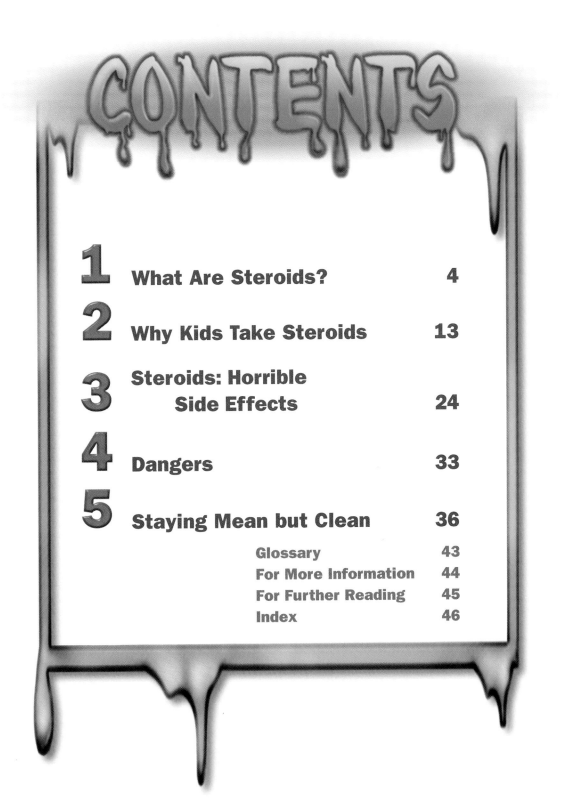

1 What Are Steroids?

Most kids your age have heard about steroids. Whether it's the Tour de France bicycle race or the Olympic Games, it seems as if you can't watch a sporting event without a steroid scandal erupting. Despite increased drug testing, evidence that steroids can be very dangerous, the risk of a ruined career, and the fact that taking steroids is a criminal offense, more athletes are using steroids and other illegal performance-enhancing drugs than ever before.

Although steroid use in professional sports receives a lot of attention, big-name athletes are not the only users and abusers. Much less talked about, but equally alarming, is the increasing number of young people—boys and

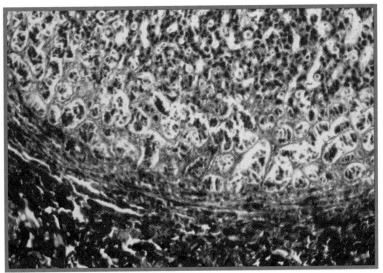

Steroids are naturally occurring hormones produced
and released by your adrenal glands (above).

girls—who use "roids," "juice," "pump," or "hype" to
make the team, win the tournament, or simply to acquire a
body that appears tough and buff.

BUT WHAT EXACTLY ARE "ROIDS"?

Everybody has steroids. They are a group of hormones that
your body produces. They are released by your adrenal glands
(which are located above your kidneys) and also by your
reproductive organs—guys' testes and girls' ovaries. Natural
steroids produced by your body are extremely important. They

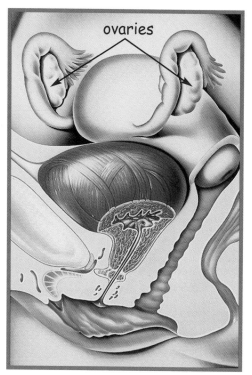

ovaries

Steroids are also released by the ovaries (above).

help to develop sexual characteristics—muscle strength, deep voice, body and facial hair, breast growth, testicles, genitalia, sperm production—and help control your metabolism. They also prevent inflammation, regulate your immune system, balance the amount of salt and water in your body, and increase your body's ability to fight illness and injuries.

STEROID USE

Unfortunately, some people have conditions or illnesses (such as asthma, arthritis, and lupus) that prevent their bodies from producing steroids. In such cases, they might need to take chemically manufactured steroids in order to stay healthy. Corticosteroids mimic cortisone and hydrocortisone, two hormones produced by the outer part (cortex) of your adrenal glands. If taken in doses that exceed those naturally made by your body, they can fight inflammation. For this reason, corticosteroids are the steroids most often prescribed by doctors for people with medical conditions.

Cortisone

Cortisone was first detected in 1935 by researchers at the Mayo Clinic. By 1948, doctors at the clinic were using the hormone to treat severe cases of rheumatoid arthritis, a condition in which a person's joints ache and swell up so much that he or she sometimes can't even get out of bed or hold a pen. This successful treatment led to other experiments and other uses of cortisone.

When cortisone was first discovered, it was viewed as a miracle drug. Doctors and patients were so enthusiastic that

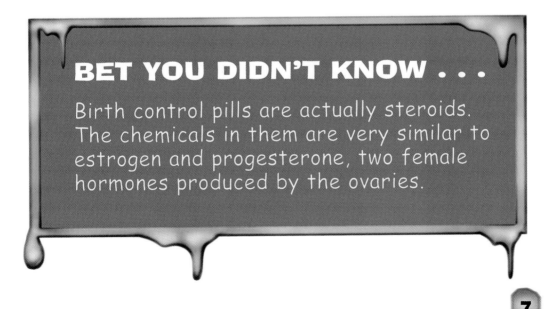

BET YOU DIDN'T KNOW . . .

Birth control pills are actually steroids. The chemicals in them are very similar to estrogen and progesterone, two female hormones produced by the ovaries.

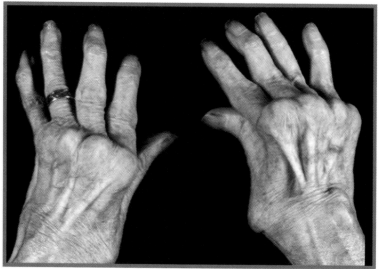

Cortisone, first identified in 1935, was used to treat severe cases of rheumatoid arthritis.

they prescribed and took extremely high doses of this steroid. Patients experienced harmful physical and psychological side effects, which in turn gave steroids a negative reputation.

Today, many pharmaceutical companies make different kinds of corticosteroid drugs, and doctors have found that lower dosages and different ways of taking the drugs (using cortisone creams, for example) have reduced many side effects. Such drugs treat conditions ranging from allergies, asthma, and arthritis to tissue diseases such as lupus and arteritis (inflammation of the arteries). People who receive organ transplants also take these steroids. Because they prevent your natural immune system from kicking in, corticosteroids help prevent the body from rejecting a new organ.

ANABOLIC STEROIDS

When people talk about steroids, they are usually referring to anabolic-androgenic steroids. Anabolic comes from the Greek word for "building" and androgenic means "masculinizing." Anabolic-androgenic steroids, commonly called anabolic steroids, live up to their name. They are responsible for the development of muscle strength and size and for male sexual characteristics, such as a deep voice and body hair. The male hormone testosterone is a natural anabolic-androgenic steroid.

Manufactured anabolic steroids were first produced in the 1930s to treat a condition called hypogonadism, which occurs when a guy's testes don't make enough testosterone. The effects of this condition range from permanent puberty to impotence. Substituting anabolic steroids for testosterone allowed guys' bodies to develop normally and to function sexually.

STEROID ABUSE

Low doses of anabolic steroids are used to treat a variety of diseases, including some types of anemia (in which a person gets very weak as a result of a lack of red blood cells), breast cancer, some kinds of impotence, and the weakening of the body caused by AIDS and other diseases. Today, there are over 100 different kinds of anabolic steroids available in North America. Without a doctor's prescription, it is illegal to use any of them. However, because steroids enhance physical performance—allowing you to lift more weights or run longer and feel less stress, for example—and help to build up your body, anabolic steroids have been used illegally by both athletes and nonathletes since the late 1950s.

How Steroids Are Taken

Steroids can be taken orally, rubbed into your skin (in cream or gel form), or injected into your muscles using a needle. The amount of steroids people use when they're trying to increase their strength is much greater than that prescribed by a doctor for medical purposes. In fact, some athletes, in a big hurry to achieve fast results, take extra-large doses of steroids known as megadoses. Although both males and females use these drugs, guys—who feel much more pressure to excel at sports or to acquire a "built" physique—are more frequent users. Steroids are especially popular among bodybuilders and weight lifters.

Cycling, Stacking, and Pyramiding

There are different ways people take steroids.

 Cycling: Taking multiple doses of steroids for a certain time, stopping for a while, and then starting again.

 Stacking: Taking several types of steroids at the same time. The steroids are chosen for the way they will interact with each other. The effects on your muscle growth are much greater than if you were only taking one kind. However, these combinations can be dangerous. It is hard to know what effect they will have on your body.

 Pyramiding: Gradually increasing your use of steroids, either by taking more and more drugs at one time or by increasing the dose and frequency of steroids taken (or by doing both at the same time). In the middle of the drug-taking cycle, the user reaches a peak amount (the top of the pyramid) and then begins to cut back until he or she reaches the end of the cycle and can begin all over again. A "cycle" can last between six and twelve weeks.

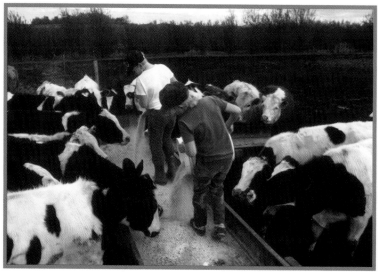
Veterinary steroids are normally used in animals and may be dangerous to humans.

While these different ways of taking steroids might not seem to pose any additional threat to your health, the irregularity with which you stop and start taking large amounts of different types of powerful drugs can create serious problems for your body and your mind. Some steroid users will stop at nothing to build up their bodies. Doses taken by steroid abusers can be anywhere from 10 to 100 times higher than those prescribed for medical problems. Some "juicers" are so desperate for mega-muscles that they mix traditional steroids with veterinary steroids, normally reserved for horses, cows, pigs, and other big animals who have hormonal problems. This is definitely not healthy, and do you really want to look like a farm animal?

2 Why Kids Take Steroids

Because taking steroids for nonmedical reasons is illegal and can get athletes disqualified or banned from sporting events, it's hard to know how many North Americans actually do abuse steroids. However, it is believed that hundreds of thousands of adults use anabolic steroids at least once a year. And the scary thing is that among adolescents, steroid use is growing rapidly, especially among young women.

Some Troubling Statistics

A 1999 survey funded by the National Institute on Drug Abuse (NIDA) tried to find out what percentage of middle school and high school students admitted to having used steroids at least once in their lives. Their findings were pretty worrisome.

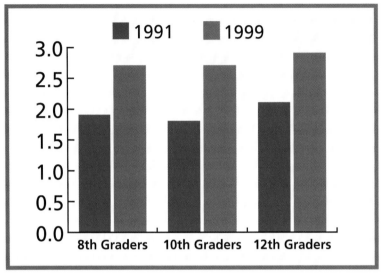

Percentage of Students Taking Steroids

■ 1991   ■ 1999

8th Graders   10th Graders   12th Graders

WHY KIDS TAKE STEROIDS

This section of the book will discuss a few of the most common reasons why young people take steroids.

To Improve Their Performance in Sports

The most common reason for steroid abuse is the desire to excel in sports. Evidence shows that anabolic steroid use promotes lean muscle mass, strength, and the ability to train longer and harder. Bodybuilders and weight lifters are the biggest users and abusers of steroids. Increasingly, though, players of other sports are using steroids, too. Contact sports (football, baseball, and wrestling, for example) that depend on players' size are seeing an increase of steroid users, as are swimming, cycling, and track and field, where endurance is important.

The Pressure to Perform

Steroid abuse is most common in professional sports where winning and losing can make or break a career. The American Heart Association estimates that at least half of all Division 1 college football players have used steroids over long periods of time. However, college football aside, in North America an overwhelming number of people— coaches, recruiters, the media, parents, and kids them- selves—are taking sports more and more seriously. Even in high school, middle school, and intramural sports, there is more pressure to perform well and to win.

In our culture, sports figures are worshiped. So is the money and success their athletic performance can bring them. For many kids growing up in tough economic circumstances, excelling at football or basketball can mean winning a scholarship to a top high school, college, or university. It can even lead to a career in professional sports and, for a lucky and talented few, to fame and fortune.

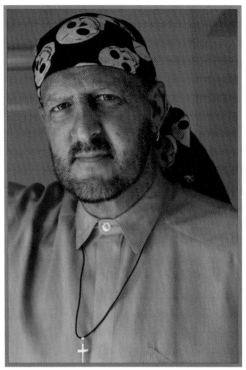

Steroids caused the brain cancer that killed NFL star Lyle Alzado.

The increasing pressure not just to do well, but to win at all costs, makes it difficult for many young athletes to say no to steroids. You may not want to take steroids, but you might worry that if you don't, you'll be at a disadvantage competing against kids who do take them. Remember the old saying "It's not whether you win or lose, it's how you play the game"? Well, society is telling kids that it is whether you win or lose, and many kids are so afraid of losing that they are willing to use steroids to win.

By the Way, Competing When on Steroids Is Cheating

It is estimated that between 6 and 11 percent of high school athletes in America use steroids. If you compete in sports and you use steroids, you're cheating others and yourself as well. Where's the triumph of winning if it is not due to your own skills? Because steroids make competitions unfair and give certain athletes (those with money and access to high-priced drugs) advantages over others, anabolics have been banned from sports since the 1976 Olympics. Since then, rigorous testing has become the norm at every level of competitive sports. Even colleges, high schools, and amateur sports leagues are resorting to drug testing. And testing is increasingly accompanied by punishments ranging from fines and suspensions to expulsions from teams.

Think that big-name athletes are untouchable? Just think of Ben Johnson being stripped of his gold medal in the 1988 Seoul Olympics. Think of Lyle Alzado, one of the NFL's star players from the mid-1970s through the mid-1980s. After he retired, Alzado admitted to using steroids, even when his doctor warned him not to. He beat his wife in a steroid-fueled rage. Steroids also caused the brain cancer that led to his death in 1992, at the age of forty-three.

As you will see in the next chapters, steroids can cause permanent physical and psychological damage. But your friends, teammates, or even your coaches may pressure you to use steroids anyway.

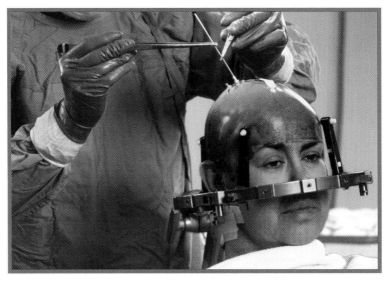

Steroids can cause brain cancer, which is what is being treated by a doctor in this photo.

Looking Good

Steroid use among teens is growing rapidly because kids want to achieve "the look"—what you see when you open any bodybuilding magazine, rent any movie with Stallone or Schwarzenegger, watch a *Baywatch* rerun, or leaf through a magazine full of ads for men's clothing or cologne. "The look" is everywhere. In the same way that, over the years, girls and women have felt pressure from society to have model-like bodies, boys and men are now feeling these pressures. The media is selling us the message that a desirable guy is one with pecs and abs and a stomach as flat as a surfboard. Though these are superficial ideals, and we may know that looks aren't everything, the pressure is still on.

Because of this pressure, many girls take diet pills and starve themselves to the point of suffering from potentially dangerous eating disorders (anorexia nervosa and bulimia). Guys are taking steroids in order to bulk up and acquire muscles. According to a 1995 study, 22 percent of American teens admitted to using steroids to improve their appearance. Two years later, that number had shot up to 38 percent. Many guys think that girls (or other guys) won't like them or find them attractive unless they have the body of a lifeguard.

Here's the Truth—Muscles Don't Matter

One of the biggest myths concerning body image is that guys think that girls go for big, bulging muscles. However, research shows that as far as girls are concerned, less is actually more. In a study where both men and women could choose the ideal male body, men chose images of bodies that, on average, were twice as big and bulky as those chosen by women. Doctors who carried out the study in the United States, France, and Austria came up with the same conclusion: Instead of wanting to bulk up to please women, men actually want to look bigger to impress other men!

19

When Fear Leads to Steroid Abuse

"I have no desire to harm other people, but until I got to 297 pounds (on a 5'9" frame), there were a lot of guys who wanted to use me as a punching bag."

—Former Mr. USA and pro bodybuilder Craig Titus

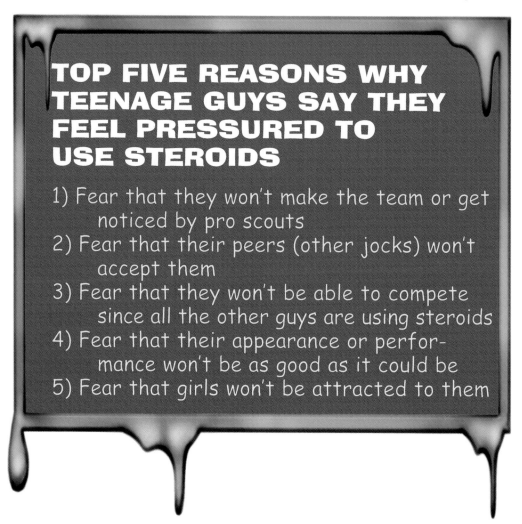

TOP FIVE REASONS WHY TEENAGE GUYS SAY THEY FEEL PRESSURED TO USE STEROIDS

1) Fear that they won't make the team or get noticed by pro scouts
2) Fear that their peers (other jocks) won't accept them
3) Fear that they won't be able to compete since all the other guys are using steroids
4) Fear that their appearance or performance won't be as good as it could be
5) Fear that girls won't be attracted to them

An increasing number of neighborhoods and school-yards in the United States are unsafe places. Increasingly, both teenage guys and girls feel physically threatened and insecure. Bulking up—especially if you're small and wiry—makes many kids feel safer and more powerful in the face of bullies, gangs, and even an abusive parent or sibling.

When Antonio's dad walked out on him, his mom, and his younger sisters, his mom said to him, "Okay, now you're the man of the house." Although Antonio was only thirteen, in his mother's culture a man is supposed to pro-tect the family no matter what. Feeling the weight of this responsibility, Antonio joined a gym and started taking steroids. For him, being a man meant looking and acting like one.

In a study of male weight lifters, 25 percent of those who abused steroids admitted to being victims of physical or sexual abuse as kids. Of those who didn't use steroids, none had experienced abuse.

MUSCLE DYSMORPHIA

Muscle dysmorphia is when a person has a distorted image of his or her body. Guys with this behavioral condition are convinced that they look small and wimpy, even if they are big and muscular. Girls with this problem feel that they look overweight even if they are actually trim and slim. People with muscle dysmorphia often use steroids: guys because they want bigger muscles, girls because they want to reduce their body fat. Sadly, no matter how many steroids they take, they will never be satisfied.

In a study of female weight lifters, victims of rape were 50 percent more likely to use steroids. Many of these women

G.I. WHOA!

Need proof of how out of proportion society's obsession with male muscles has gotten over the years? Just take a look at G.I. Joe. Scaled to human size, the original 1965 plastic action figure had biceps with a circumference of 11.5 inches—more or less that of your average American male. By 1995, the plastic he-man was sprouting biceps of twenty-six inches—larger than any bodybuilder in history!

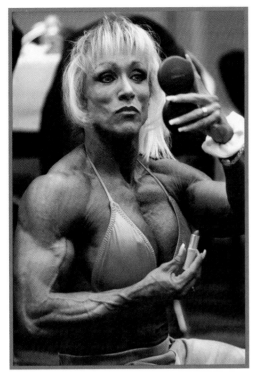
Some rape victims use steroids to develop "masculine" bodies.

wanted to toughen up and be stronger, but they also hoped that if they developed masculine bodies, men would see them as ugly and intimidating and would not consider trying to sexually abuse them.

As you can see, in an overwhelming number of cases, teens abuse steroids out of fear—fear of not winning; of not living up to the expectations of parents, friends, team-mates, or society; of not being attractive; or of not being able to physically defend oneself.

In a few cases, teens abuse steroids simply because the risk excites them. Just as some adolescents get a thrill from drinking and driving too fast, taking heavy drugs, or not wearing a helmet on a motorcycle, some young people choose to use steroids because they like to flirt with danger.

3 Steroids: Horrible Side Effects

Many drugs have negative effects on your mind and your body. What many people don't know is that steroids can mess with your emotions, too. Some of these effects are temporary; if you stop using steroids, they will go away. However, other side effects are permanent.

The scary thing about steroids is that while studies have been done about the short-term effects of steroids, little is known about long-term effects. If some of the problems described in this chapter sound horrible to you, imagine how bad they could become over a longer period.

PHYSICAL EFFECTS

Even if used only for a short time, steroids can produce all sorts of undesirable and dangerous problems. Sure, your muscles will increase and your body fat might decrease. But as you continue to use more steroids over time, you could also begin to experience muscle cramps, aching joints, nosebleeds, nausea, vomiting, diarrhea, insomnia, trembling, and water retention. At the same time, while your muscles might swell to Herculean proportions, you are also a likely candidate for severe acne and jaundice, a condition where your skin, tissues,

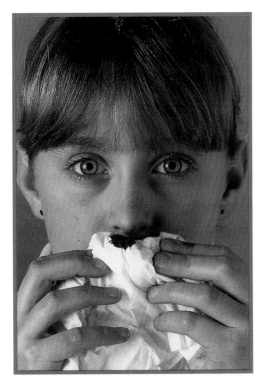

Steroid use causes nosebleeds and other gross side effects.

body fluids, and even eyes turn yellow. If you can't quit shaking, and you're all yellow and covered with zits, you're not likely to impress anyone—no matter how muscular you are.

If you think that these general side effects are a small price to pay for using steroids, read on to see how steroids can affect both guys and girls. One thing that

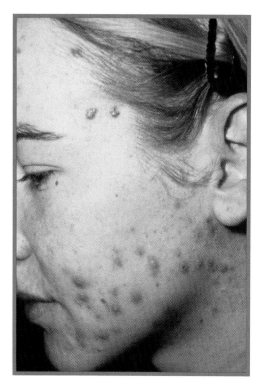

Steroid use can cause acne.

could happen is that your muscles and tendons—the tissues that connect your muscles to other parts of your body, such as your bones—may begin to tear. This is likely to occur because anabolic steroids weaken tendons.

The Awful Things You Can't See

With steroid use, many damaging changes take place inside the body and these things may not be noticed until it is too late. People who abuse steroids have a higher risk of experiencing serious life-threatening conditions that range from high blood pressure, high cholesterol, infertility, and a weakening of the immune system's defenses to osteoporosis (disintegration and cracking of the bones), liver, heart, and kidney diseases, heart attacks, and many serious forms of cancer. Although some of these effects are reversible—if you stop taking steroids, they will eventually

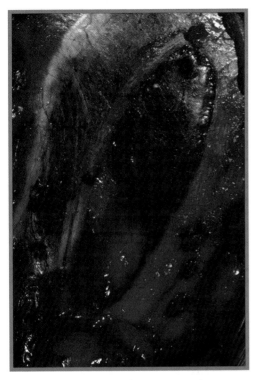

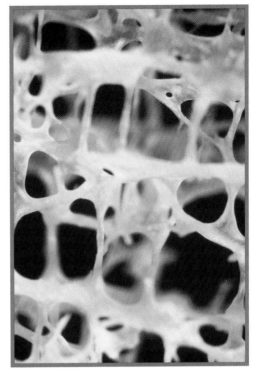

Anabolic steroids can weaken tendons such as these.

Steroid use can cause osteoporosis, a weakening of the bones.

disappear—others, such as the growth of hair on your face and the deepening of your voice if you're a woman, are irreversible, meaning that they will last forever.

"When I was thirteen, I was still the smallest guy in my class. All the other guys were bigger and more muscular. They treated me like a little kid, called me "shrimp-o," and were always picking on me. I was always the last to be

chosen for any sports team. I was so miserable that I had to do something. So I started taking steroids. I took a lot because I was in a big hurry to grow up.

At first it seemed as if they were working. Suddenly, I shot up and bulked up a bit. But just when things got going, they stopped. Later, the doctor told me that the roids had forced my body into puberty before it was ready. My own hormones never kicked in because of the roids. So today I am 5'2" and my doctor says I won't ever grow any taller. I regret what I did to my body."

—Bobby, eighteen years old

PSYCHOLOGICAL EFFECTS

It has been proven that steroid abuse, particularly in high doses, can cause severe mood swings, which can lead to extreme aggressiveness and violent acts. This is so common that it is known as roid rage. Roid rage has led some steroid abusers to get into fights, commit armed robbery, or destroy property. People who take steroids are more likely to hurt themselves or others.

Steroid users can also experience panic attacks, para-noia, extreme jealousy, severe irritability, and hallucinations (when you start seeing or imagining things that aren't there). Mania (an extreme hyperactive high), depression, and psychosis are other possible side effects. Needless to say, all of these can have a very negative impact on your relationships with family members, friends, boyfriends, girlfriends, teachers, etc. You risk creating a lot of personal problems and alienating yourself from those who care about you.

Using steroids makes some people feel as invincible and untouchable as Superman or Wonder Woman. Not only does this lead to taking not-so-smart risks, but it also can cloud your sound judgment in many matters.

"I really believed that I was a goddess or something. When I remembered how skinny I was before I started using steroids compared to a year after . . . I could lift so much weight. I looked great in the mirror. The other girls on the track team, they seemed to be jealous of how I looked. I would never have thought that steroids would one day turn against me—that I would be constantly shaking, that I'd tear the tendons in my leg and not be able to run, that I'd start doing all this crazy stuff like beating up my little brother in a sudden rage for no reason at all."

—Jackie, fourteen years old

ADDICTION

One of the most common problems associated with steroids, and the most difficult to treat, is mental addiction. After all, once you've experienced the strength and weight increase that steroids produce, it's hard to stop taking them. Steroids can give you a false high or sense of confidence. Coupled with this, athletes are afraid that their performance will suddenly slide. Other people are afraid of looking the way they used to, so they keep using and abusing steroids, often in increasingly dangerous quantities. Before they know it, they're completely addicted.

When you're addicted, you want to keep taking more steroids, which increases the already serious health risks (not to mention that steroids are costly). Being addicted means it's difficult to quit. Teens who do try to get off steroids will often experience withdrawal symptoms, including mood swings, feeling tired or restless, insomnia, and a lack of appetite.

Depression

The most frequent and serious consequence of addiction is the depression experienced as users feel themselves "losing their power." This depression can make it especially

HORRIBLE SIDE EFFECTS OF STEROID USE

Guys

- Your testicles will shrink
- Your sperm count will plunge
- You'll be infertile
- You'll go bald
- You'll grow breasts
- Your prostate will grow, with an increased risk of prostate cancer

Girls

- You'll experience stunted growth
- You'll have irregular periods
- You'll grow hair on your face and body
- Your voice will get deep and manly
- Your breasts will shrink

hard to stop taking steroids. In some cases, it is so severe that it can lead to suicide attempts. If left untreated, depression can last for a year or more after a person stops using steroids. If you or anyone you know is addicted to steroids, and you fear that he or she may be depressed, speak to an adult you can trust, and get help.

(VERY) EARLY ADOLESCENCE

Accidental contact with a steroid cream caused a North Carolina boy to enter puberty at the age of two!

Over a four-month period, the young child sprouted pubic hair, broke out in pimples, and grew a penis that measured three inches. All of this because his dad was using a testosterone muscle-building cream. Whenever the boy was held or hugged by his father or crawled around on his dad's steroid-covered bodybuilding mats and equipment, he came into contact with the steroid.

Once the problem was discovered, and the contact with the steroid was stopped, most of the boy's acne and pubic hair disappeared. His penis, however, remained the same size.

4 Dangers

Apart from the side effects caused by the actual drugs themselves, there are many other dangers involved with steroid use.

NEEDLES

One of the most common ways of taking steroids is by injecting them directly into your muscles with a needle. Users—particularly teens—often use needles given to them by friends, dealers, or other drugs users. It is hard to know where a needle has been, but the risk of injecting steroids into your body via a conta-minated needle is very real.

Frequently, needles are shared or stolen. One popular way of getting needles is to find out which students or friends' parents are diabetic and steal their needles. Although it sounds pathetic, rifling through these people's garbage bins is more common than you would think. However, what's really dangerous is that shared, stolen, or scavenged needles can be contaminated with a number of viruses. Two of the most serious are hepatitis, which causes serious damage to the liver, and HIV, which leads to AIDS.

FAKE STEROIDS

Because using steroids without a prescription is illegal, steroids are bought and sold on the underground market. As this is illegal, there is no way of controlling the quality of the steroids. Like any other hard-core illegal drug, steroids may have been exposed to unsafe substances and surroundings. More than likely they are fakes or counterfeits.

Many of the most popular steroids, both real and fake, are easily available in Mexico. Smuggling them across the border to the United States has created a thriving drug business. Many of these steroids are black-market imitations that are ineffective, or they are made in clandestine (secret) laboratories in filthy conditions—meaning that the drugs are often contaminated with impurities or bacteria. It has been estimated that close to 90 percent of black-market steroids are contaminated or are mixed with unknown substances.

In the United States, making counterfeit steroids is a big business. Labels are made to resemble those on legitimate drugs. These illegal steroids are transported and sold through networks of drug traffickers, just like, and along with, other types of illegal drugs. Pushers don't care about the origin, safety, or quality of what they are selling. They often even sell low-quality veterinary steroids that were never meant to be taken by humans. Pushers just want to make a fast buck from addicts who will buy the juice no matter what.

It's a Crime

Since 1990, when Congress passed the Anabolic Steroids Control Act, possession or sale of steroids for nonmedical reasons has been a crime in the United States. This means that if you do take steroids, you'll not only have to worry about immediate side effects and future health problems, but about the legal consequences as well. Most kids have no idea what could happen to them if they are caught breaking the law.

The laws are tough, and so are the consequences. Being caught with steroids is the same as being caught with a vial of crack. An upstanding young student found with steroids will be considered a felon and will risk going to jail. Obviously, this can seriously affect not only a sporting career but any kind of professional career you plan to undertake.

5 Staying Mean but Clean

Steroids are not chemically addictive. This means that unlike some other hard drugs, your body does not crave them or need them. If you quit taking steroids, your body will not miss them. Instead, steroid users develop a mental addiction. Users are convinced that they have to have them to look good, feel strong, and perform well. They convince themselves that they can't live without steroids. The difficult side effects, mostly depression, that hit when a person stops taking the drug make quitting even more difficult.

GETTING OFF STEROIDS

Although surprisingly little research has been done to establish effective treatment for steroid abuse, doctors recommend therapy. Users are taught about what to expect during withdrawal and are monitored for severe depression or suicidal thoughts. If withdrawal symptoms are serious or last a long time, medications might be prescribed. These could include drugs that restore your hormonal balance (steroids interrupt the body's natural production of these), antidepressants for treating depression, or analgesics for headaches and muscle pain. In extreme cases, hospitalization might be necessary.

If you were or are taking steroids because of an image problem—you feel weak, unattractive, insecure—or if you are or were a victim of physical or sexual abuse, seek counseling. Talk to your parents, your coach, your guidance counselor, your family doctor, or any other adult you trust. Together, try to find a counselor or therapist who can help you deal with your problems. Taking steroids is not a solution. It can really harm your body, and it is against the law. However, admitting that you're using is nothing to be ashamed of, especially if you need help and want to quit.

STEROIDAL SUPPLEMENTS

You might have heard about how in 1998, the year he set a new home-run record, baseball player Mark McGwire

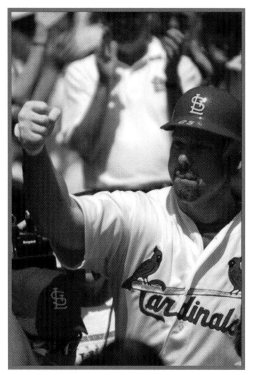

Mark McGwire used andro to help him set a new home-run record.

was taking a steroidal supplement called androstenedione (known on the street as "andro"). The thing about andro and other steroidal supplements, such as DHEA and creatine, is that they can be purchased legally (without a prescription) in places such as health food stores. Although they are often referred to as dietary supplements, steroidal supplements are taken because users believe that they have anabolic effects. In the body, these drugs are converted into small quantities of testosterone. Whether enough is produced to create big muscles or to increase strength is unknown. However, some abusers take massive quantities, hoping that the combination will help them beef up or improve their game.

Less is known about these "supplements" than is known about steroids, and for this reason, they are

ONE DRUG LEADS TO ANOTHER

Recent research suggests that steroid abusers are more likely to abuse other hard drugs, particularly heroin. Many steroid users are introduced to such drugs by the same dealers who sell them roids. Some start taking heroin to deal with the insomnia and irritability caused by steroids. Others get hooked when they try to get off steroids and find themselves depressed.

potentially very dangerous. Although they are not yet illegal, many sporting and government organizations are categorizing them as anabolic steroids. For a start, they have been banned by the National Football League, the National Collegiate Athletic Association, and the International Olympic Committee.

Although McGwire stopped taking andro and still played a great season in 1999, a frightening number of kids (an estimated 5 percent of middle school and high school athletes) have admitted to taking creatine. While it might make muscles bigger, short-term effects include dehydration, muscle cramps, and possible kidney failure. Long-term effects are unknown but threaten to be even more serious.

SAFE ALTERNATIVES TO STEROIDS

People are always looking for an easy solution or a miracle drug. Although steroids might appear to be both of these things, they're not. Steroids cannot make you a better athlete. They won't make you more agile or increase your skills. The famous saying "It sounds too good to be true" sums up steroids perfectly.

Steroid abuse can cause kidney disease.

If you aren't satisfied with your body or with your athletic performance, there is only one way to make a positive improvement: through hard work. There are no shortcuts. The following are surefire secrets to success. Of course, if you think about it, you'll realize that there's nothing secret about these hints. They are incredibly straightforward:

 Talk to your coach/trainer (make sure he or she is a professional) and work out a safe training routine.

 Stick to your training schedule.

 Do a variety of activities that you enjoy and that work different parts of your body.

 Eat a healthy well-balanced diet. Don't resort to fad diets or food supplements.

 Don't smoke or drink alcohol.

 If you're bodybuilding or weight training, get a professional to supervise your activities.

 Get plenty of sleep and take time to relax.

 Set realistic goals and reward yourself when you reach them.

 Play safe and use protective equipment in order to avoid injury.

ADOLESCENTS TRAINING AND LEARNING TO AVOID STEROIDS—ATLAS

Funded by the National Institute on Drug Abuse (NIDA), ATLAS is a recently developed program that uses positive peer pressure to help fight steroid use in schools. Originally, the program was developed for male football players and their coaches. It consists not only of classroom discussions and debates (no lectures or preaching) but also weight training taught by specialized trainers. Sessions deal with the negative impact of steroids, but they also focus on alternatives such as sports nutrition and strength training techniques. Decision-making and drug-refusal skills are practiced as well.

Because of its open, nonjudgmental nature, ATLAS has been really successful. After completing the program, 50 percent of teens quit using steroids and another 50 percent decided they would never try them. Since the program is expanding, it is now being tailored to help kids on any kind of sports team—both guys and girls—as well as teens who use steroids simply because they want to be more muscular.

GLOSSARY

anabolic   Building.

androgenic   Masculinizing.

cycling   Way of taking steroids in off and on cycles.

hypogonadism   When a male's testes don't make enough testosterone.

impotence   When a male can't get an erection.

inflammation   Result of an injury to a cell or tissue, characterized by redness, heat, and swelling.

jaundice   Condition in which your skin, tissues, and body fluids turn yellow.

paranoia   Extreme feelings of fear or mistrust.

pyramiding   Increasing dosage or frequency of steroids to a high point and then decreasing.

stacking   Taking various types of steroids at the same time.

tendons   Tissues that connect your muscles to other parts of your body.

testosterone   Hormone responsible for male sexual characteristics.

FOR MORE INFORMATION

In the United States

American College of Sports Medicine (ACSM)
401 W. Michigan Street
Indianapolis, IN 46206
(317) 637-9200
Web site:
http://www.acsm.org

National Institute on Drug Abuse (NIDA)
U.S. Department of Health and Human Services
601 Executive Boulevard, Room 5213
Bethesda, MD 20892
(301) 443-1124
(888) 644-6432
Web site:
http://www.nida.nih.gov

Partnership for a Drug-Free America
405 Lexington Avenue, Suite 1601
New York, NY 10174
(212) 922-1560
(800) 662-HELP (4357)
Web site: http://www.drugfreeamerica.org

In Canada

Canadian Centre for Ethics in Sport (CCES)
2197 Riverside Drive, Suite 300
Ottawa, ON K1H 7X3
(613) 521-3340
(800) 672-7775
Web site: http://www.cces.ca

Canadian Centre on Substance Abuse
75 Albert Street, Suite 300
Ottawa, ON K1P 5E7
(613) 235-4048
Web site: http://www.ccsa.ca

FOR FURTHER READING

Balcavage, Dynise. *Steroids*. New York: Chelsea House, 1999.

Brouwer, Sigmund. *Chief Honor (Lightning on Ice)*. Dallas: Word Books, 1997.

Clayton, Lawrence. *Steroid.* Rev. ed. New York: The Rosen Publishing Group, Inc., 1998.

Kuhn, Cynthia, Scott Swartzwelder, and Wilkie Wilson. *Buzzed: The Straight Facts About the Most Used and Abused Drugs from Alcohol to Ecstasy.* New York: W.W. Norton and Co., 1998.

Miklowitz, Gloria D. *Anything to Win*. New York: Delacorte Press, 1989.

Monroe, Judy. *Steroid Drug Dangers.* Springfield, NJ: Enslow Publishers, 2000.

Peck, Rodney G. *Drugs and Sports.* New York: The Rosen Publishing Group, Inc., 1998.

INDEX

CREDITS

About the Author

Albert Spring is a trilingual journalist. He has a twin sister named Annie.

Photo Credits

Cover and p. 27 right © Michael Klein/Peter Arnold, Inc., cover inset by Cindy Reiman; p. 5 © A. & F. Michler/Peter Arnold, Inc.; p. 6 © John Bavosi/Science Photo Library; p. 8 © National Medical Slide Bank/Custom Medical Stock Photo, Inc.; p. 12 © Richard Hamilton Smith/Corbis p. 16 © Neal Preston; p. 18 © Roger Ressmeyer/Corbis; p. 23 © Wide World Photos; p. 25 © Victor De Schwanberg/Science Photo Library; p. 26 © Biophoto Associates/Science Source; p. 27 left © M. English/Custom Medical Stock Photo, Inc.; p. 38 © AP/Wide World; p. 40 © OJ Staats/Custom Medical Stock Photo, Inc.

Series Design

Laura Murawski